Action Guide

By Wendy Ida

FOREWORD BY LES BROWN

Motivational Speaker
and Bestselling Author

The Take Back Your Life Action Guide

Wendy Ida is available as a keynote speaker for expos, conventions, seminars, workshops and other media events. For more information or for additional copies of this book, please contact Wendy Ida Enterprises at: info@wendyidafitness.com

Cover photo by Jurgen Reisch

Layout and interior design by Joanne Shwed, Backspace Ink, Pacifica, California (www.backspaceink.com).

First printing

ISBN: 978-0-615-54176-1
Published by Wendy Ida Enterprises Inc

Printed in the United States of America

Dedication

I dedicate this Action Guide to all of you who have the courage to stare fear in the face and take action right here and right now towards your ultimate goals. For those who are a little reluctant, I'm praying that you keep the faith and push beyond your doubts and fears, no matter what age you are or what state of being you may be in …

Acknowledgements

Thank God for his strength, comfort, guidance, life lessons and the courage to face life's uncertainties.

I give many thanks to Randy Peyser and Gail Martin for their assistance, knowledge and support throughout my book projects. You are simply the best! Most of all I thank and appreciate my family for their love, support and patience.

Contents

Foreword

You Deserve Good Health

An introduction by motivational speaker and bestselling author, **Les Brown**

For more than two decades, I have traveled the world helping people learn to live their dreams. But how can you live your dreams to the fullest if your health is compromised? It's absolutely clear to me that good health is not a given, you have to work for it. You deserve good health. When you are in good health, you have the stamina to go the distance, to do what it takes to win. When you're not in good health, everything becomes more difficult.

I've often said that "a lot of people are content with their discontent." Too often, people put up with things they don't like because it's easier that way. They pretend not to notice, even though they're still not happy. That kind of thinking is not going to help you live your dream. It's not going to help you win. And if you're discontented with your health-whether you're overweight, have diabetes, have no energy for living, or whatever the problem-you're being held back from that dream. As a 15-year cancer conqueror I can attest that many people have overcome serious illnesses to go on to achieve great things. But how many more great things could they have achieved and how much easier would it have been for them to achieve those goals had they been in good health?

I want you to live your dream. So when Wendy Ida asked me to introduce Take Back Your Life, I understood that Wendy made the connection between good health and achieving one's dreams. Wendy has overcome negativity and tragedy because Wendy had the hunger and courage to change her life. And when she took action and made those changes, she found a way to empower other people.

Wendy's "OWN" system of "Outlook, Workout and Nutrition" requires a commitment on your part, but I've always said that once you make a commitment, then life will give you some answers. Even more than that, learning to *Take Back Your Life* by taking the steps you need to take to improve your health will enable you to overcome whatever is keeping you from reaching your dreams.

I believe with all of my heart that you have it in you! You have the discipline and drive to live your dreams. And I also believe that you have the self-love and motivation to improve your health. You deserve good health.

Take your life in a new direction; develop new relationships with people that are positive, healthy and fit, and full of life and energy. The *Take Back Your Life* program will require that you make the decision that you want to live. You may need to change some old habits of negative thinking or to change beliefs that are holding you back. That's the price of attaining good health. You may need to change eating habits that are working against you and making you unhealthy. So be it. You may need to change your daily routine to get off the couch and up on your feet to strengthen your body and lift your mood. So get up! Get up now! Get up and shout to the world that you are going to

Take Back Your Life! I know that change is difficult. But I also know that change is essential for survival. And Wendy and I want you to do more than just survive. We want you to thrive!

Maybe you feel like you have hit a wall when it comes to your health. Perhaps you've had a major setback, a serious illness, or an ongoing challenge. Maybe you've gone through a divorce or lost your job, or have become a caregiver and it's taken the fight out of you. None of this is an excuse to give up. It's not a reason to become "content with your discontent." You deserve good health. So if you've hit a wall when it comes to getting healthy, reach out to someone on the other side of the wall who can help you climb over the wall. Let Wendy Ida be that person for you. Wendy will help you get out of your unhealthy comfort zone. She will show you how to eat better, how to see possibilities, and how to build strength and stamina so that when the opportunities open up for you to live your dream, you are ready to go the distance.

I believe that you deserve good health. I want you to experience the blessing of being healthy, but more than that I want you to eliminate all of the obstacles that stand between you and your dreams. And if your health is an obstacle to achieving your dreams, then you need to change your health. Wendy's T*ake Back Your Life* system will show you how to overcome the Outlook, Workout and Nutrition challenges that are holding you back and set you free to grow. You have within you the power to achieve your dreams. I believe that, and so does Wendy Ida. Now it's your turn. It's time to *Take Back Your Life* and turn your dreams into reality.

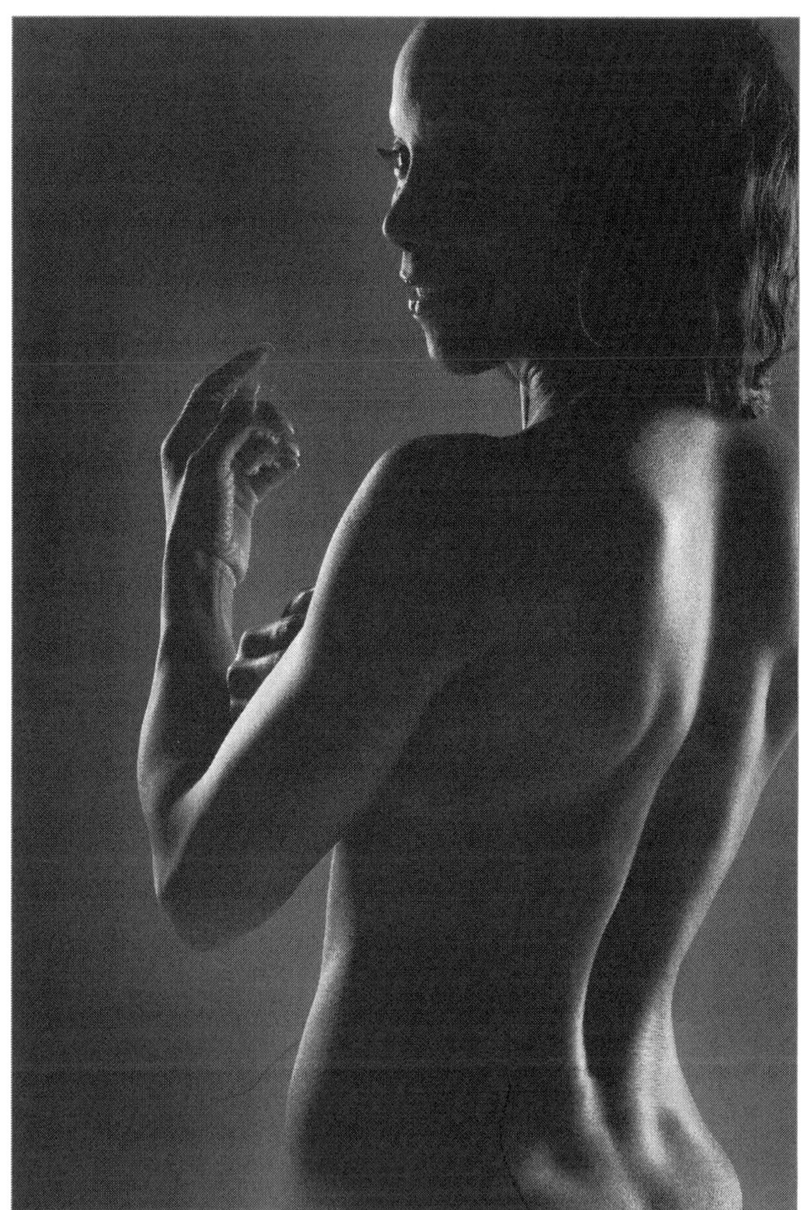

Introduction

Welcome to *The Take Back Your Life Action Guide*. I've designed this Action Guide as a guided journal specifically for YOU, so you can personalize the *Take Back Your Life* book and create the spectacular results you want.

This guided journal is your companion on the exciting journey that lies ahead of you. Big changes often happen a little at a time. Sometimes, it's difficult to see the big change you're making until you look back.

Please use this journal to record your feelings as you *Take Back Your Life*. Journaling will enable you to review how your thoughts and feelings change throughout your transformation. And of course, writing down your feelings will help you to work through any rough spots you encounter along the way.

I want to encourage you to use this *Action Guide* to explore these questions:

- How did I get to this point in my life?
- Why do I want to change?
- What do I want to change?
- What do I expect from the change I want to make?
- How might I be holding myself back from making those changes?

- What success am I seeing in making the changes I want to make?

Please think about this *Action Guide* as a companion journal, a private place where you can have a conversation with yourself. Use the journal to record your thoughts and feelings without fear of judgment, like talking to a trusted friend. You can revisit the pages as you see changes in your life unfold, to remind yourself of how far you've come, or to motivate yourself to keep moving forward.

I hope this *Action Guide* becomes your favorite companion on your amazing journey to *Take Back Your Life*. Changing your Outlook is an essential part of your transformation, so the thoughts you record and the shifts in thinking that you honor here in this journal will play an important role in your overall success. I'll be with you all the way—with questions, quotes, and more to keep you excited and engaged.

Your journey to *Take Back Your Life* is the most important thing you can do for yourself and for the people you love. Always remember that you're not alone. I'm here supporting you through the pages of this *Action Guide*, cheering you on. The people who love you are rooting for your success, too. You can do it! I believe in you!

Love,

Wendy

CHAPTER ONE

Midlife Motivation Hurdles

What have been some of your best accomplishments? These can be personal (such as raising children or renovating a home), professional (degrees, promotions, success on the job) or spiritual (like dealing with abuse or dysfunction, finding forgiveness for yourself or others, etc.) List as many as you can:

....

....

....

....

....

....

....

....

....

How can you use what you've learned from these past successes and accomplishments to help you Take Back Your Life with your Outlook, Workout, and Nutrition goals?

....

....

....

....

....

....

....

Aside from losing weight or getting in shape, what would make you feel sexy? (Be honest! List your turn-ons, such as a sexy nightie [or nothing at all!], champagne and soft music, a special location, perfume, or anything else you can think of.)

....

....

....

....

....

....

....

What kinds of things can you do every day to make yourself feel sexy and special? (For example, wearing sexy undies, splashing on perfume, dressing up a little more, wearing high heels, etc.)

....

....

....

....

....

....

When you feel sexy and special, how does it affect your mood? Your can-do attitude? How you feel about your ability to reach your goals?

....

....

....

....

....

....

"I think the quality of sexiness comes from within. It is something that is in you or it isn't and it really doesn't have much to do with breasts or thighs or the pout of your lips."
—Sophia Loren

Motivation Mind Game #1—Remember When

Remember the last time you had a great workout? How did you feel? Were you energized, upbeat and really proud of yourself? Did it help you sleep better? Did it make you feel sexier? Was it a prelude to great sex? Write your answers here and revisit them when you need a boost!

....

....

....

....

....

....

....

Motivation Mind Game #2—Let's Make a Deal

When you're tired and not in a work-out mood, figure out a 'deal' you can make with yourself (it shouldn't involve food!) to get you to go to the gym. For example, telling yourself you'll only do eight reps instead of twelve, or thirty minutes on the treadmill instead of forty-five. Of course, when you get there, you'll often feel good enough to go beyond the bargain. So—what's your 'deal' to get yourself motivated on the days when you don't feel like doing it?

....

....

....

....

....

....

....

Motivation Mind Game #3—The Buddy System

Exercise is more fun with a friend. Make a list of all the people you could invite to different types of workouts, and make a note of what kind of exercise might be the best fit. For example, a work friend might be up for taking a walk on lunch break. Another friend might prefer Yoga in the evening, while someone else might be an early morning gym buddy. Make your list here—and add phone numbers so you've got no excuse about calling!

....

....

....

....

....

....

CHAPTER TWO

OWN Your Outlook

The power to change comes from realizing that you control you. That's right. YOU control YOU!

Who are your role models or heroes? These can be famous people, or the friends, relatives, teachers, leaders and others who made a big positive impact on your life. Write down their names here, and beside the name, a word or two on what makes them your hero.

....

....

....

....

....

....

....

....

....

Faith plays a big role in being able to OWN your Outlook. Whatever your beliefs, take a moment to write down a short prayer, affirmation, intention or mantra that will help to motivate and inspire you. (Keep it positive—no guilt or negatives!)

....

....

....

....

....

Revisit your list of role models and heroes. Think about the famous names on your list. How much do you know about their struggles and what they overcame to succeed? Promise yourself that you'll check out a biography about one of your heroes from the library this week. Not a reader? Look for a show on the Biography Channel on TV, or download a show about your hero from Netflix or the Internet. Make a note of the important things you learned about your hero's struggles and successes here:

....

....

....

....

....

Create your 'board of directors.' Mentally, picture the heroes and role models who are important to you. Make them real in your mind. Imagine that you can talk to them—and hear their replies. Now, ask your heroes for advice on whatever problem you face, and let the things you've read about them come back to you as if they were speaking just to you. Listen to their wisdom and ask them to encourage you. Make a note here of what you've asked, who answered, and what your 'board members' recommended.

....

....

....

....

Find your talisman. Your talisman is something you can touch or hold to remind you of what your dreams are. It could be a charm on a bracelet or necklace, a smooth rock in your pocket, or a picture by your computer. When you are tempted to give up or feel 'stinking thinking' sneaking back into your mind, touch your talisman to keep yourself on track. Choose your talisman and write down why you chose it.

....

....

....

....

Name your dreams. Getting fit, learning to eat right, and losing weight are great dreams. What other dreams do you have for the rest of your life? Speaking your dreams aloud and writing them down are two powerful ways to help your dreams become real. Take a moment to write down your dreams, big and small. Then sit in a private place and read the list out loud. Make time to do this every day, or at least several times a week.

....

....

....

....

Build your vision board. A vision board is a type of talisman because it helps your dreams stay real. Take a piece of cardboard or foam board. Cut out pictures from magazines or the Internet of the things you want most. If you want a family, choose a picture of a happy couple with children. If you want to travel, choose pictures from the places you want to go. Carefully arrange the photos into an attractive display on your board and then place it where you will see it frequently. Write down your thoughts about the pictures you chose. Why were those photos special? What do you think when you see them? Be specific about the dreams the photos represent so that you don't forget.

....

....

....

....

Strength and growth come only through
continuous effort and struggle."
—Napoleon Hill

CHAPTER THREE

Using the Delta Factor and Omega Attitude to Achieve Your Goals

Use your Delta Factor

There are five sections in the Delta Factor: Fuel, Activity, Strength, Flexibility, and Stress Reduction. Cultivate all five and you have a strong base to help you succeed as you Take Back Your Life.

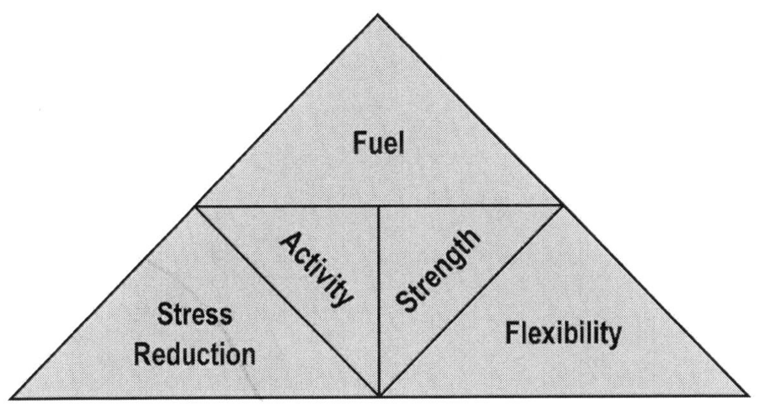

Fuel — How are you going to fuel your effort to Take Back Your Life? Good food is one way. Getting at least eight hours of sleep is another. But fuel also comes from heroes and role models, friends and family who cheer you on, and the positive mental messages you give yourself. Take a moment to jot down how you will fuel your journey.

....

....

....

....

....

Activity — Sure, you're active in the gym, but the Delta Factor goes beyond the gym. How can you work more activity into your daily life? Can you take the stairs, walk the dog, mow the yard, rake leaves, or play ball with your kids? What other 'activity' are you making a priority in order to Take Back Your Life? Are you reading or watching biographies of your heroes? Consulting your mental 'board of directors'? Saying your dreams aloud? Using your talisman and vision board? Make a list of all the activities you're doing to make your dreams come true.

....

....

....

....

....

Strength — Increasing your weights at the gym is one kind of strength (good for you!). But you'll also need mental strength to overcome old habits. Go back to the list of activities you made above. Which of those activities will help you gain strength to beat bad habits and stay on track?

....

....

....

....

....

Flexibility — Flexibility is important at the gym to avoid injury, but it's equally essential outside of the gym. When your day goes crazy (and it often will), how can you be flexible and still stay true to your goal to Take Back Your Life? If you can't make it to the gym, can you walk or work out at home with DVDs and simple equipment? If you're traveling and can't have exactly the food you need for your nutrition goals, how can you substitute to do as little damage as possible?

....

....

....

....

....

Stress Reduction — Stress sneaks up on you, and if you're not prepared for it, stress will sabotage your progress. Working out or taking a walk can help burn off stress. Meditating, doing Yoga, listening to music and other calming activities can help you regulate your feelings. What are your favorite stress busters? List them here, and come back to this list the next time you're stressed out.

....

....

....

....

....

Creating your Omega Attitude

The Omega Attitude has three elements: Confidence, Creativity, and Consistency. You'll need all three to Take Back Your Life.

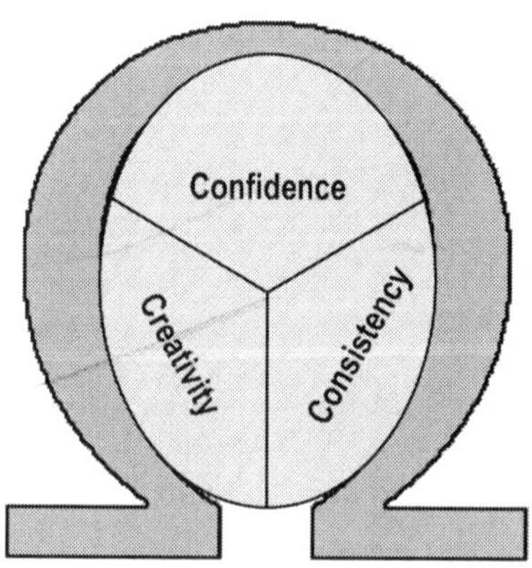

Confidence comes from knowing you can win and achieve your goals. It also means believing that you deserve to win. Create your own set of confidence statements and use them the next time you need a dose of Omega Attitude.

- I believe I deserve to Take Back My Life because . . . .
- I know I can win my battle over . . . .
- I believe I can achieve my goal to . . . .
- I deserve to live the life I've dreamed about, which includes . . . .

Add your own statements here:

....

....

....

....

....

....

....

....

....

....

Creativity keeps you motivated. It helps you learn, play, and grow. Creativity can mean different things to different people. Cooking, writing, sewing, doing crafts, playing music, drawing and painting, sculpting, acting, and singing are just a few ways people show their creativity. What are your favorite creative things to do? Make a list, and promise yourself you'll fit one of your favorites in for at least a few moments every day.

....

....

....

....

....

....

....

....

Consistency means you stick with your plan even when the going gets tough. Hang a calendar in your kitchen, and buy yourself three different kinds of fun stickers. Make it a little ritual to go to the calendar each day before you go to bed. Give yourself one sticker if you've worked out. Put up another sticker for making the effort to eat nutritiously. Use the third sticker for keeping your Outlook on track. Now take a moment and look at the other days with stickers. Congratulate yourself for being consistent! Look at the days to come. Picture yourself being consistent tomorrow and the day after that. You can do it!

....

....

....

....

....

....

....

....

"The most essential factor is persistence—the determination never to allow your energy or enthusiasm to be dampened by the discouragement that must inevitably come."
—James Whitcomb Riley

CHAPTER FOUR

Food Strategies

Playing some mind games with yourself can help you stay on track to finish what you started. Being in control when you eat, while you eat, and where you eat is the goal here.

Banish temptation — Make a list of your food favorites, the foods you have difficulty controlling. Get them out of your house—and don't buy them anymore. Write your list here to remind yourself what not to buy.

....

....

....

....

....

....

....

....

Share food gifts — When someone gives you a food gift, share it and pass it on! Take it to work, bring it to a neighborhood get-together, or leave it in the break room. Think about the people and occasions where food is a likely gift and make a list of what you can do to dodge the pudge!

....

....

....

....

....

....

....

Staving off cravings — When you've got the urge to eat and you're not really hungry, what actions can you take to distract yourself? Here are some of my favorites: Get up and move around; leave the area where the food is; drink several glasses of water; chew gum. Now, make your own list. Think about the most common times you're tempted to eat when you aren't hungry, and match a distraction to each time!

....

....

....

....

You can also Take Back Your Life by actively looking for foods that will boost your mood, decrease stress, and improve healing. Start your search on the Internet, and then seek out books about healing with food. Ask your doctor, nutritionist, or alternative practitioner for suggestions. Then look for ways you can incorporate those healing foods into your recipes and daily diet. Journal on the following:

- My list of foods that can help me to heal:

....

....

....

....

....

....

....

....

- My list of foods that can help decrease stress:

....

....

....

....

....

....

....

....

- My list of foods that can help me to boost my mood:

....

....

....

....

....

....

....

....

"Freedom and life are earned by those alone who conquer them each day anew."
—Johan Wolfgang von Goethe

CHAPTER FIVE

The Take Back Your Life Basic 90-Day Plan

Affirmations help you to keep your Outlook on track. An 'affirmation' is a statement of belief or positive self talk that helps get you out of a slump and keeps you focused. Now it's time for you to create some affirmations of your own.

Step One — Look at my list of example affirmations in Chapter Five if you have the *Take Back Your Life* book. Write down the ones that really speak to you here:

....

....

....

....

....

Step Two — Now create your own affirmations. Make as long a list as you want. Here are some starter phrases:

- I will . . . .
- I can . . . .
- I am . . . .
- I deserve . . . .
- I commit . . . .
- I know . . . .

Create your own guided meditation. In Chapter Five, I explained how you can use guided meditation as a quick pick-me-up when you're stressed, or a way to unwind. A guided meditation is a story that you walk through in your mind, a journey that puts you in a peaceful and safe place where you feel loved and confident.

Go back and read through my guided meditation in Chapter Five of the book. Yours can be longer or shorter, but it should be a journey that really speaks to you.

> "I deserve (fill in the blank). I deserve (fill in a different blank). (Action) and (action) are helping me Take Back My Life. I am confident of (fill in the blank). I am (fill in an action you're taking to achieve your goal). I am (fill in the accomplishment you are achieving). Working out makes me feel (fill in the blank). Eating well makes me (fill in the blank). I feel healthy and sexy. I like what I see in the mirror. I have the power and knowledge I

need to Take Back My Life. Every day I take another step toward accomplishing my goals. I feel great!"

Another type of guided meditation helps you relax by giving you a mental vacation. Choose images that invoke all of the senses, so that you can imagine taste, sight, smell, touch, and sound. Your guided meditation may take you back to a place you've been that was special to you, or to someplace you've only dreamed of going. Here are some ideas to get you started.
Picture yourself walking down a path toward a peaceful place. Imagine walking down a set of steps to your sanctuary—a secluded beach, a quiet forest, a garden—whatever appeals to you. Imagine the sounds that you would hear in this quiet place. What are the scents in the air?

Think about how this place affects all of your senses. Now in your imagination, find a place to sit in this sanctuary where you feel comfortable and safe, a place where you would like to linger for a while. Imagine that you have no pressing deadlines, no reason to hurry, nothing to do except enjoy this peaceful place. How do you feel?

Stay in your sanctuary for as long as you want to do so. Soak up the warm sun, or refresh yourself in the shade. Listen to the sounds around you, feel the breeze on your skin, take in the calming scents. Marvel at the beauty all around you. As you enjoy the sanctuary, feel yourself growing more refreshed and relax. Notice how your body and mind let go of tension. You can come back to your sanctuary whenever you need a break from the pressure of the world outside.

When you're ready to leave, say a mental 'thank you' to the beauty all around you. Remember that you can come back whenever you want to. Take one last deep breath, and then make your way back to the steps and climb back up to the 'real' world. How do you feel?

CHAPTER SIX

Maintaining Your Outlook When Life Changes

Big changes in your life can derail your mood, interrupt your workout, and throw your nutrition off track. To Take Back Your Life when circumstances throw you a curve ball, you'll need to set your intentions and take control.

How is your current situation affecting your life in these ways:

- Your workout?

....

....

....

....

....

- Your ability to eat healthy food and healthy portions at regular intervals?

....

....

....

....

....

- Your ability to sleep soundly and to get enough sleep to feel rested?

....

....

....

....

....

- Your ability to cope with stress in positive ways?

....

....

....

....

....

Changing circumstances can also change your perception of yourself. You may find a change in what you want from life, what you expect from yourself and what you need from others.

- What major life changes have happened to you in the last twelve months?

....

....

....

....

- How are these changes affecting how you see yourself and what you want?

....

....

....

....

- Do you view these changes as negative or positive? Why?

....

....

....

....

When life changes, your Delta Factor is more important than ever. Your ability to feel empowered no matter what life throws at you begins with your intention to take control.

Beside each of the following Delta Factor elements, write down ideas about how you can honor yourself and your commitment to Take Back Your Life by finding a way to work each of these into your daily routine:

- Fuel (physical, mental, and spiritual food):

....

....

....

....

....

....

- Activity:

....

....

....

....

....

....

- Strength:

....

....

....

....

....

- Flexibility (physical and mental):

....

....

....

....

....

- Stress reduction (physical and mental):

....

....

....

....

....

....

Now, think about how the Omega Attitude can help you deal with your changing life circumstances. What ideas do these three components spark for you so you can put them to use and Take Back Your Life?

- Confidence:

....

....

....

....

- Creativity:

....

....

....

....

- Consistency:

....

....

....

....

Gratitude is an essential element for positive transformation. It can be difficult to find gratitude during trying situations, especially when change is painful. Yet there are small things in every day to feel grateful for: a bird outside the window, the sun, a child's laughter, the touch of a friend, even a good cup of tea.

Create a 'gratitude log' of the things (big and small) you find each day that you can feel grateful for. Begin your journal here:

....

....

....

....

....

When chaos strikes, affirmations can help you remain focused on your intentions. Affirmations are short, positive sentences that speak about your goals for the future. For example, one affirmation you might want to use is: "I will surround myself with positive influences today to keep my energy high." What affirmations can you claim to help you stay on track?

....

....

....

....

....

Don't waste time and energy second-guessing yourself over things in the past. 'Woulda,' 'coulda,' and 'shoulda' are three words that cause a lot of problems. Banish them from your vocabulary and your thoughts! What old baggage are you ready to let go of so that you can stop looking back with regret and start looking forward with excitement?

....

....

....

....

....

"If there is no struggle, there is no progress."
—Frederick Douglass

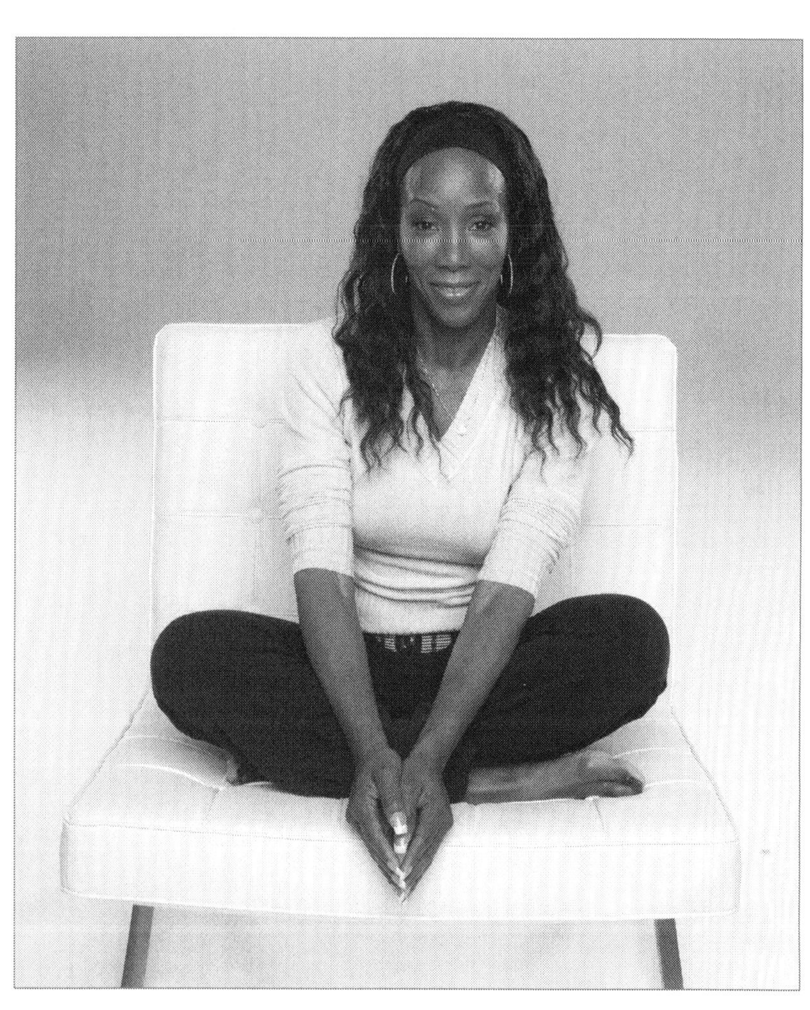

CHAPTER SEVEN

Creating a New Life When Relationships Change

As we move through life, our relationships change. Divorce, Empty Nest Syndrome, Grief, and Care-giving are inevitable stages of life. As your world changes, it's important to focus on caring for yourself, finding whatever positives you can in a situation, and look for reasons, even in the midst of sadness, to be grateful for what you still have.

During any time of loss (and changing life circumstances often feel like loss even when good things later come of them), meditation is essential for growth. Meditation is an element of that Delta Factor Fuel, as well as a proven stress reducer. You don't need anything fancy, and meditation doesn't have to be religious. Something as simple as breathing can be a start.

Here are some easy ways to meditate. Try them out, spending about five minutes with each exercise. Make a note of how you feel, and which approaches work well for you.

Breathing — Sit somewhere quiet and comfortable where you won't be disturbed (don't lie down if you're likely to fall asleep). Close your eyes, and focus on the simple process of breathing in and breathing out. Feel your breath come in, then let it go. If you're stressed and breathing shallowly, try to slow down your breathing until your in-breath and your out-breath are even and longer. Feel your whole body relax as you focus on the sound of your breath, the beating of your heart, the rise and fall of your chest.

Notes:

....

....

....

....

....

Affirmative phrases — Think of a word that has positive connotations. 'Peace', 'comfort,' 'strength,' 'blessings,' 'insight,' and similar words can all work well. If you are a religious person, you might think of a short phrase like "God is with me," or "Give me strength, Lord." Keep your phrase short and positive. Now, find a quiet place where you can close your eyes for a few moments without interruption. As you breathe in, think your phrase. Let the phrase be in tune with your breath. Now, repeat the phrase as you breathe out. Do this for several cycles, in and out.

Notes:

....

....

....

....

....

Visualization — Sit somewhere quiet and close your eyes. Be comfortable. Now, imagine a golden light touching you on the top of your head. It is warm and comforting and healing. Very slowly, the light works its way down from the crown of your head to your forehead, your mouth, into the muscles of your neck and shoulders, and on down your body until it reaches your toes. Visualize the light moving down your body, saying to yourself, "As the light reaches my (shoulders), I feel warm and relaxed." Say each area of the body that the light touches as you visualize it, and focus your attention on relaxing that part of your body.

Notes:

....

....

....

....

....

Which type of meditation worked best for you? How did you feel when it was over? How can you make time for the meditation you chose in your daily schedule? Write your thoughts here:

....

....

....

....

....

Ask for help when you need it. Going through a major life change is difficult. You don't have to do it alone. Don't let your pride get in your way! There are many people who care about you, and trained helpers who will support you in a kind and caring way, even if you are meeting them for the first time. Asking for help when you need it is a positive step toward your goal to Take Back Your Life.

What kind of help would make it easier for you? (Be specific and make a wish list. Don't worry about 'how' or 'who' just yet.)

....

....

....

....

....

Look over your list. Where could you go to find out what options for help are available? How can you get in touch with someone who can help you make connections? Who do you know with the skills to provide some of the help you need?

....

....

....

....

....

Accepting help is the next step to Take Back Your Life. Many times, caring people offer help but we're too proud to accept it. It's okay to accept help. If you're in crisis, don't worry right now about how to pay your helper back. Often, it's enough to know that, in time, you will 'pay it forward' and extend a similar helping hand to someone else in need in the future.

Who has offered help? What have you done about the offer? Would the help that has been offered make your situation easier? What is keeping you from accepting the help?

....

....

....

....

....

Too often, we allow shame or the fear of judgment to keep us from asking for or accepting help. Yet truly helpful people will not judge you or make you feel guilty. They just want to help you get through a rough spot. Think about accepting the help that has been offered. How does it feel? Accepting help should make you feel better. If you imagine yourself feeling guilty or beholden, try to figure out why. Banish those negative thoughts. You're not Superman! It is normal and healthy to ask for and accept help when you need it.

When our relationships change, we often let the change affect our own self-worth. Are you telling yourself negative things about yourself because of the change in your relationship? If so, write down those things here:

....

....

....

....

....

....

....

Now, look at the list of negatives. These are the hurtful things you have been telling yourself. But are they really true? Think back to other relationships you have had that were positive and healthy. Remember how you felt about yourself then. Write a list of some of the ways you felt positive about yourself in the past.

....

....

....

....

....

....

....

Now go through your negative list again, and replace each negative with one of the positive feelings you have felt about yourself. Whenever you start to put yourself down, replace the negative thought or feeling about yourself with one of the positive words you've added in this journal entry:

....

....

....

....

....

....

....

Stress from relationship changes can torpedo your nutrition and healthy eating habits. When people are uncomfortable, they often eat out of boredom or stress, and not because their bodies actually need the food. And when people are stressed, they don't usually pig out on salads! During this time of stress, eat for fuel and strength, but be mindful of the times when you're tempted to eat out of stress and boredom. In the space below, make a list of the times when it's tempting to eat when you don't need the food, and find a substitute activity (reading, taking a walk, going to the gym, cleaning a room, etc.) that you could do instead.

....

....

....

....

....

....

A change in your relationship status can give you more free time. Some people over-commit to social activities or volunteer work because they are afraid to be alone. Others are frightened by their newly free schedule and retreat or hide. Neither extreme is healthy. Think about how you could spend your new free time in ways that help you achieve your goals, move you closer to your intent to Take Back Your Life, or make you happy. Make a list of those activities here, and refer to them when you're feeling at a loss as to what to do.

When your relationships change, you change. Whether you're experiencing a loss from divorce or grief, or going through a transition from Empty Nest or Caregiving, you are becoming a new and different person. You are not on a quest to Take Back Your (old) Life, but to Take Back Your (power to live your new) Life. This is a time for reinvention! List all the ways you can think of that you could reinvent yourself if there were no limits. Be silly, be extravagant, be outrageous. Free your imagination without censoring yourself.

Now look carefully at your reinvention possibilities to find out exactly what your passion is. What do you absolutely love to do? What makes you feel alive? What would you do even if no one paid you? What gives you joy? Think about how you could reinvent yourself to give yourself more of that joy, love, passion, and sensation of life. Write down your ideas here:

....

....

....

....

....

....

Sometimes a makeover in one area leads to new beginnings in another area. As part of your reinvention, consider updating your look. Change your hair style or your hair color. Buy a new outfit. Have your makeup done at a department store or by a professional. For a small investment, you'll get a whole new lease on the way you feel, and the pick-me-up of having a fresh start. Write down what you've done to update your look, and how it makes you feel. Add your 'Before' and 'After' photos, weight changes and measurements in the sample forms at the end of this Action Guide to help you remember how far you've come!

....

....

....

....

....

....

Whether your relationship change has given you more free time or less, how about rethinking what you cook to spice up your creativity? Eating the same things night after night or week after week gets tiresome. Healthy eating is fuel and strength, and it can be fun, too! Go online for some new recipes, pull out a cookbook, or pick up a recipe card at your local grocery store and try something new!

If you're used to cooking for more or fewer people, look for delicious recipes to fit your current situation. Show yourself love by planning and preparing tasty and healthy meals for yourself. Make a list of the new meals you're discovering, or of recipes you want to try. Or if you don't cook, where can you find healthy meals and fresh ingredients?

....

....

....

....

....

....

When a relationship changes or someone we love moves on without us, it can be difficult to imagine life 'after'. Yet, life goes on, the sun will rise, and believe it or not, good things (even great things) lie in store for you. Don't let yourself get stuck in the past, and don't feel guilty about looking for good in the future. Take Back Your Life! Make a list of at least five good things you hope will become part of your life over the next few years.

....

....

....

....

....

It's essential to come back to gratitude as you move through your journey to Take Back Your Life. You will be grateful for different things and to different people as your journey progresses. As you move from loss and chaos into positive action, you will 'wake up' and begin to see the world around you with fresh eyes. Make a list of all the things and people you are grateful for right now, at this stage in your journey.

....

....

....

....

....

When we're in the midst of relationship changes, including grief and chaos, it can feel as if we are surrounded only by bad things. Yet there is good all around us, even if we can't see it clearly. When we notice the good, it uplifts us and gives us hope. Set your intention to find two or three good things each day, and write them down.

These could be positive things that happen to you, beauty that you see in the world around you, or good things that happen to others or that you read about happening elsewhere. Train yourself to start looking for good things, and you'll begin to see goodness in the most unlikely places! Start your list here:

....

....

....

....

....

When we are hurt, we tend to pull back. Yet there is a wide and wonderful world waiting for us to re-engage with it. We begin to re-engage by being mindful, by being present in the here and now. Pull yourself out of your thoughts and fears with mindful breathing, as I've described earlier.

Now that you are 'here,' use your senses to reconnect with the world around you. Walk in a garden. Kick your feet in a pool. Listen to the wind in the leaves overhead. When you're ready, find a social activity with a nurturing group of people and attend it. Don't judge yourself. What can you do to reconnect with the world around you? List your ideas here.

....

....

....

....

....

Sometimes, when changes in our relationships throw us into chaos, we get so busy taking care of others or taking care of tasks that we stop taking care of ourselves. To Take Back Your Life, you must make time for yourself! If that thought seems overwhelming, think of small steps to fit into your daily schedule. Beside each suggestion below, write your own thoughts, ideas and ways you can fit self-care into your situation right now.

- Meditation

....

....

....

....

....

- Exercise (even ten minutes at a time makes a difference)

- Flexibility: Stretching, Yoga, Tai Chi, etc.

- Enjoying nature (watching birds at a feeder, sitting outside for a few minutes, going for a walk, etc.)

- Reading a book that inspires or gives you pleasure (even if it's only a few pages at a time)

- Calling, emailing, or 'Facebooking' a friend for a quick chat

- Fixing a healthy meal

- Getting enough sleep

....

....

....

....

....

- Spending a few minutes (or more) doing a hobby you enjoy

....

....

....

....

....

- What can you add?

....

....

....

....

....

In some relationship changes, isolation is part of the transition, especially when you're keeping vigil in a hospital or nursing home, or you are alone in a new place. Yet there are always people around us, even if you don't recognize them as 'people' because of the role they play. The nurse at the front desk of the hospital ward, the orderly who cleans up the room, the cashier at the coffee shop, the mailman, and others often move through our lives like ghosts we don't really see.

Try greeting each 'invisible' person in your daily routine with a cheery smile, a friendly hello, and an upbeat comment. You'll be amazed at how strangers turn into friends, or at least, into friendly acquaintances you'll look forward to seeing. Make a list of the 'invisible' people in your life, and jot down what happens when you begin to greet them, chat with them and thank them.

....

....

....

....

....

"When you are content to be simply yourself and don't compare or compete, everybody will respect you."
—Lao Tzu

CHAPTER EIGHT

Navigating Career Changes

Whether you are leaving a job by choice or not, career changes bring on stress and upset your daily routine. It takes a while to settle into a new 'normal'. That's true whether you are retiring, changing jobs, recovering from a layoff, relocating, or adapting to a promotion. Accept that it will take a while for you to settle in, but keep your commitment to Take Back Your Life by finding ways to remain on track.

Use the gift of time. If you are between jobs, newly retired, or adjusting to life after a layoff, you've got a new and somewhat blank schedule in front of you. Resist the urge to fill it from morning to night in order to distract yourself from the discomfort of change. Instead, think about the ways you can use some of this free time to reduce stress, reach your fitness goals, or just relax before diving into what comes next.

What could you do with the gift of time that you've been given? List at least ten activities that would be healthy, enjoyable, and/or help you adapt and relax.

....

....

....

....

....

....

Seize the opportunity to use this time of change to make a real transformation. Now that you have a little leeway in your schedule, what can you do to create the New Professional You? What do you envision as the new and 'improved' you? Make some notes here to capture your thoughts.

....

....

....

....

....

....

Now's a good time to look back at the job you just left. Think about the best parts and the worst parts, so that your next role will have more of what you want and less of what you don't want. This is also part of the Take Back Your Life approach, because a job you hate is one of the biggest stressors in your life. Get the job you deserve!

What did you like best about your previous role? (Things you'd like more of in the next job.)

....

....

....

....

....

....

What did you hate about your last job? (Things you want to avoid in your next role.)

....

....

....

....

....

....

What aspects of your last job contributed to an unhealthy mind or body? (Stress, toxic people, crazy schedule, pressure, no downtime, etc.)

....

....

....

....

How can you assure that your next role is healthier?

....

....

....

....

When you're in a time of career transition, making positive workout and food changes can be a great way to feel more in control of your situation. Not only that, but making positive changes now to Take Back Your Life means you'll be in tip-top shape to start that new role! What will you do to use this time to create healthier workout and eating changes?

....

....

....

....

Career transitions can be hard on the ego. You no longer have the old title or status that you were used to having. The people around you have changed. Whatever perks your job had are gone. During these transitions, it's all too easy to mentally beat yourself up. Stop it! Your mental dialogue is crucial to being able to Take Back Your Life.

You need positive self-talk and affirmations. List ten things you can tell yourself to keep your thoughts positive and focused on the great things that are going to come to you!

....

....

....

....

Today, people can 'retire' from one career and create another, jump from a corporate life into a role as an entrepreneur, take a time-out from work to pursue education or a life-long passion, or choose to end their working careers and retire in a traditional way. Regardless of which type of 'retirement' you choose or experience, you'll need some new goals to go with your new life. Goals are essential for you to Take Back Your Life and retain a sense of meaning and purpose. List your new goals here:

....

....

....

As you build your new life, make sure to leave room for the things you love. Hobbies are more than just a distraction; research shows that people who are passionate about causes or hobbies live longer than those who don't have pastimes they enjoy. If work or your family life have crowded out hobbies that you used to enjoy, or if you've never had the spare time to indulge a passion, now is the moment! What hobbies or passions do you want to explore?

....

....

....

....

....

....

Career transitions are also a great time to think about giving back to the community. Volunteering will provide a wonderful networking opportunity for you to meet and connect with new people. It's also a great way to help you get your mind off of your own situation and any temporary discomfort you might be feeling by focusing on helping others. There are volunteer and community service opportunities for every schedule and taste. Some opportunities are even available online! Where can you put your skills, interests, and heart to good use helping others?

....

....

Make your workout your anchor during this career transition. Your exercise time can be an oasis—a place where you don't have to think about anything more than keeping up with the pace of the music or counting your weight reps. It can become the constant in your newly fluid schedule. Make sure your workout is a mixture of cardio, strength training, stretching, and some routines that encourage better balance. In addition to the Take Back Your Life workout program, explore the options available within your own community for dance, cycling, Yoga, Pilates, hiking, running, or team sports. Check out the YMCA, local gyms, recreation centers, and other community groups for great opportunities to keep your workout interesting and meet new people. What would you like to try and where can you explore your options? Make some notes here.

Food choices on the job often focus more on being quick than being healthy. Now's the time to make a change. Try some new recipes and take a few moments to chop up fresh fruits and vegetables. Reset your idea of portion sizes from large restaurant servings back to healthy quantities. What kind of food choices and changes can you make with your new schedule?

....

....

....

....

....

Sometimes, career transitions lead us to new places. That may involve retirement or relocation, a job in a different part of town, or a new role that requires travel. Whatever the reason, being in new places can be a great way to spice up your commitment to Take Back Your Life. Here are some ideas as to how to turn new locations into health opportunities. Make notes and add your own ideas!

....

....

....

....

....

Outlook – Explore new places, meet and connect with new people, see new sights. Your ideas?

....

....

....

Workout – Try guest privileges at new gyms, experiment with routines you can do in your hotel room or hotel gym, find exercise options (like walks or hiking) that can be done anywhere. Your ideas?

....

....

....

Nutrition – Discover new foods and new recipes, try new food preparation styles, explore regional or cultural dishes. Discover new 'super foods' you haven't tried before, and bring home the best new ideas as a part of your new and improved eating choices! Your ideas?

....

....

....

What foods make you feel at home wherever you eat them? Make sure you bring them with you into your new life, even if only for special occasions. If your new role takes you away from home or your home territory for long periods of time, think about how you can find some of your favorite (and healthy) comfort foods on the road. Lighten up traditional favorites by using skim milk, less butter or oil, and make other good-for-you updates.

What are your taste-of-home favorite foods? List them here, then go online for healthy recipe ideas.

....

....

....

....

....

....

Making a career transition can be exhausting, even if everything is going well. Stop and breathe. Remember the meditations and mindful breathing techniques I've shared with you, and make them part of your everyday Take Back Your Life practice. When you feel yourself moving too fast, feeling pressed for time or sinking into overwhelm, stop, breathe, and be mindful in the moment. You can do this anytime, anywhere. What makes you feel inundated and stretched too thin?

Career changes affect our social circle as well as our paychecks. When you leave a job or company, change careers, or relocate or retire, the people you've seen every day are no longer part of your daily routine. It's common to feel isolated, lonely, or alone.

Reframe those feelings of loss and get excited about the new friends and colleagues you haven't met yet. Be prepared to take the initiative to meet new people, join groups, and get connected. If you've moved to a new place, this effort will include your non-working time as well as your on-the-job connections.

How can you make an effort to meet new people? Where can you go to connect?

People are creatures of routine. We take comfort in doing pretty much the same thing in the same way every day. Even on vacation, most people fall into familiar habits. If you've gone through a career transition, your daily routine may be completely disrupted.

This can leave you feeling adrift, uncomfortable, edgy, and out of sorts. But this is also an invitation to Take Back Your Life by creating a new routine. I've listed the main components of a daily routine below. Go ahead and fill in how you'll invent a healthy, nurturing new pattern of your own that helps you create the life you want!

- Workout
- Meals
- Evening activities
- Weekend activities
- Holiday and special event activities
- Daily recurring patterns—commuting, shopping, rebuilding your social web of doctors, dentists, other health professionals, household helpers, etc.

Sex! Career changes can play havoc on your sex life. Stress, new daily routines, lack of sleep, and other side effects of your new work life can mean you're too preoccupied to be in the mood. Don't let your career change derail your intimate relationship!

Take Back Your Life by committing to make bedroom frolicking part of your must-do plan. If you have to make a date in order to see your significant other for a romp in the hay, then make an appointment! Actually put it on your calendar. Use your new schedule and flexibility to build in some 'couple time'. Take a class together, go dancing, take a nightly walk—whatever it is that brings you closer to each other.

How can you rev up your sex life with your new schedule?

....

....

....

....

....

....

....

"Choose a job you love, and you will never have to work a day in your life."
—Confucius

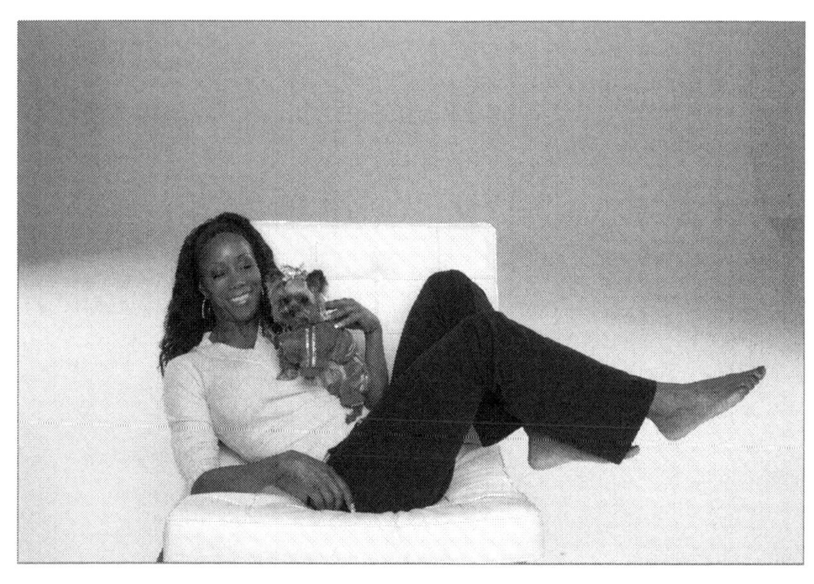

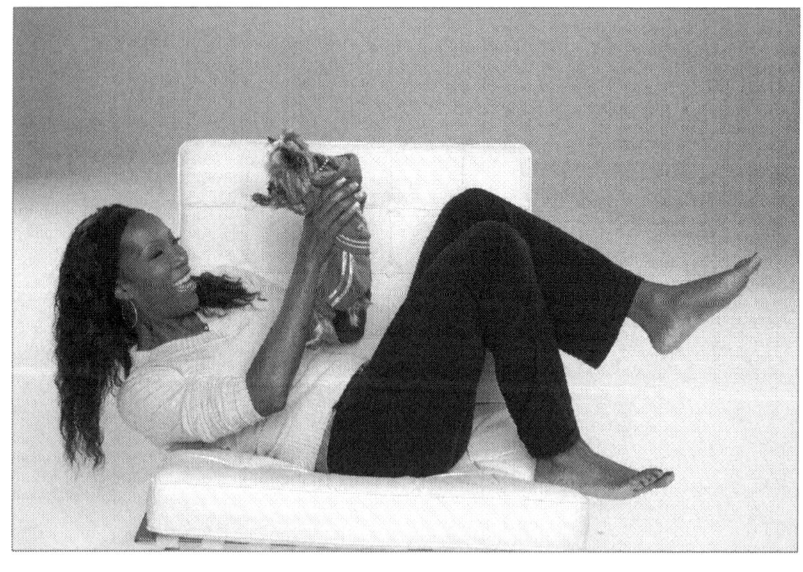

CHAPTER NINE

Dealing with Health Challenges

Nothing is more likely to derail your best attempts to OWN your future than an illness or injury. It never fails that just when you're on a roll, something happens that breaks your routine. Whether your health challenge is temporary, like a broken bone or a bout of the flu, or longer-term (like a chronic condition), you can still Take Back Your Life and find the Outlook, Workout, and Nutrition routine that's right for you.

What are your concerns regarding your health condition? Have you discussed them with your doctor? What are the doctor's instructions of activities to avoid? Did the doctor have suggestions of safe activities?

....

....

....

....

What impact does your condition make on your food choices? How can you make healthy choices within these constraints?

....

....

....

....

....

....

How does your medical condition affect your mood? Do you know how your medications may affect both mood and energy levels? Make a note here so that you can remind yourself when you are in a funk.

....

....

....

....

....

....

Have you officially entered menopause? (Your doctor can tell with some simple blood work, although perimenopause symptoms can exist for years beforehand.) Menopause is different for every woman. What symptoms are you experiencing that you associate with menopause? How do they affect your Outlook, Workout and Nutrition?

....

....

....

....

....

....

How is your health condition or the beginning of menopause affecting your sexuality? How do these changes make you feel about yourself? About sex? About your partner? About your body?

....

....

....

....

....

....

The Delta Factor is Fuel, Activity, Strength, Flexibility, and Stress Reduction. You'll need each of these elements to come back safe and strong from a health challenge, and to adjust to the changes of menopause with confidence.

Fuel — Your body has different food requirements with your current situation. What are some healthy choices you can make within the guidelines of your condition?

....

....

....

....

Mental attitude is part of your fuel. How can you reward yourself (without food), and pump up your confidence as you manage your health changes? Name at least five things.

....

....

....

....

Activity — Unless you're required to stay in bed, activity helps with mood, stamina, and weight loss. Even if your condition places limits on activity, make the most of what you are able to do. Walking is a great activity for lifting your mood, cutting your appetite and increasing endurance. Best of all, you can do it with a friend!

What activities will be a good fit for your current health situation? How will you work them into your calendar on a regular basis?

....

....

....

....

Strength — Many health conditions limit weight-bearing exercises. During menopause, hot flashes and bloating may leave you feeling blah. But studies show that even light resistance training can reduce the risk of osteoporosis, build muscle tone, and help you maintain strength.

What are you permitted to do? What do you feel able to do? Make a list of ways you can use isometric exercises, resistance bands, or light hand weights to avoid losing ground.

....

....

....

....

Flexibility — A physical injury or recent surgery may limit your options for stretching, but your doctor can advise you as to what you can do safely. If you're in menopause, realize that your body may not always move with the same ease and flexibility as it has in the past due to hormonal changes. Experiment and go slowly, never forcing yourself. Gentle programs like Yoga or Pilates can be very good to maintain flexibility without damage.

Make a list of what kinds of stretches you will incorporate into your routine to suit your current situation.

....

....

....

....

....

....

Stress reduction — If you've been ill or injured, your stress can go through the roof due to pain, doctor visits, hospital stays, uncertainty over outcomes, etc. Medication can also increase or decrease your perception of stress. During menopause, hormonal changes can play havoc with your perception of stress.

The good news is that most stress reduction requires no physical activity at all—it just needs you to shift mental gears. Here are some of my favorite ways to decrease stress—jot down ideas next to each one of these ideas that you can use as your own personal stress busters.

- Listening to music
- Going for a walk
- Enjoying nature
- Reading a book, looking at pictures
- Calling a friend or visiting with friends

- Meditating
- Taking a hot bath or a cool swim
- Playing with a pet
- Enjoying a hot cup of tea and a few moments of silence

Your Omega Attitude plays a big role in bouncing back from health conditions. Confidence, Creativity, and Consistency will guide you through this transition phase to help you emerge better than ever.

Your Confidence can take a hit when you don't feel good, or when hormonal changes leave you feeling topsy-turvy. It's important to remember that you are the same person inside that you were prior to the problem that has thrown you for a loop.

Here are some exercises to help you remember all the reasons you have to feel confident in yourself.

- Think back over the last few months. What are your biggest achievements? Or what are you especially proud of? How have you overcome challenges in the past?

....

....

....

....

....

- Remind yourself that you have overcome tough times before. When you think about the rough situations you have made it through in your life, what got you through it? Who helped you? What internal reserves did you tap?

....

....

....

....

....

....

- Find at least one thing each day that you can compliment yourself sincerely on having achieved or having done well. No matter how small, recognize and celebrate each of your personal triumphs.

....

....

....

....

....

....

Creativity will be essential as you come back from your health challenge or find your 'new normal' after menopause. If you're no longer able to do some of the things you used to do, how can you find new alternatives to explore and enjoy?

- What have you always wanted to try but didn't have the time for? Might something from that list replace an activity that you can't do now?

....

....

....

....

....

....

- What creative solutions can you find if you have new dietary restrictions or medication interactions? Can you explore new foods and new cooking techniques to discover exciting new favorites? A nutritionist can be a good source for food options that are both healthy and yummy.

....

....

....

....

....

....

- If you can no longer work out in a way you used to enjoy, what are some new options that are suited to your health concerns or to the changes menopause is making to your body? If you need help, talk with a trainer or physical therapist for good ideas.

- Your Outlook may require extra creativity to keep your sunny side up during a time when your body seems to be fighting against you. What are some creative ways to brighten your mood, or perhaps some favorite things you haven't done for a while that can turn a gloomy day around?

Consistency is the key to success. Even if you've had to make some adjustments to keep your Outlook positive and had to make changes to your Workout and Nutrition, the key to achieving your goals lies in working your plan consistently.

If your health issues force you to miss time at the gym or create a temporary upset with your food choices, get back on track as soon as you can safely do so. Picking up with as close to your old routine as possible will brighten your mood, and creating a new routine will give you a sense of structure when everything around you is changing.

You can create consistency by developing habits in the following areas. Draw a circle around the ones you like, and feel free to add ideas of your own.

- **Outlook** — practice meditation or an active mood-brightener on a regular basis. Actively seek things to be grateful for. Try to be 'mindful' by being present in the moment (instead of worrying about the past or future). Create positive phrases (affirmations) to encourage yourself. Journal and talk to supportive friends. Your ideas?

....

....

....

....

....

- **Workout** — Decide where to go, what to do, who to go with, and how often to do your routine. Your ideas?

....

....

....

....

....

- **Nutrition** — Cook and prepare food at home. Shop for food. Plan healthy meals. Choose healthy alternatives when you eat out. Your ideas?

....

....

....

....

....

Affirmations are positive phrases that help you stay focused on your goals and that enable you to keep your mind focused on health, gratitude, and wholeness. Affirmations aren't magic; however, they put the power of your mind to work for you.

Many studies have shown that people who are optimistic and hopeful tend to recover more quickly, live longer, and perceive themselves as happier than those who are pessimists. What you dwell on affects your health, your relationships, and your life! Take Back Your Life by taking back your thoughts.

You can create your own affirmations. Choose a short phrase like "I can feel health and healing radiating throughout my body," or "Forgiveness and gratitude are flowing through me." Spend a few minutes a day repeating these affirmations out loud to your self.

When you get discouraged, repeat them some more. Gratitude is also a proven mood-lifter. Combine your affirmations with statements about things for which you're grateful. For example, you could say something as simple as "I am grateful for the flowers in my garden." Now it's your turn!

Make a list of at least five affirmations that have a strong personal meaning for you.

....

....

....

....

....

Now list at least five things for which you are grateful.

....

....

....

....

....

Even with the best of intentions, sometimes your Outlook can take a nosedive. On those days, you need an EMP—Emergency Mood Plan. Have a designated friend whom you can call when your mood hits rock bottom. Identify some all-weather places where you can take a walk for a change of scenery. Create a playlist of music that makes you happy, or better yet, that makes you put on your boogie shoes! Buy a book of quotations or create your own list of motivational quotes. Find funny videos on YouTube (my favorite) and laugh. Count your blessings.

Now it's your turn—what will you include in your EMP?

....

....

....

....

....

When you're recovering from health challenges or coping with menopause, you may find yourself doubting that you're still the same sexy siren you've always been. Remember—most of sex is mental!

Here are some ideas for putting yourself 'in the mood' or just reminding yourself that you're still a sexual being and that sex is part of a healthy life. Buy some pretty lingerie or a naughty nightie. Make a romantic candlelight dinner for your significant other, or order take out and light candles anyhow. Put some romantic music on and snuggle on the couch. Go for a walk and hold hands. Pretend you're a teenager again—'make out' with your partner and try not to go 'all the way' (bet you can't resist—and if you can, you haven't been at it long enough!)

Here's your turn to list some ideas that appeal to you:

You CAN Take Back Your Life regardless of changes to your body caused by illness, surgery, or menopause. Make up your mind to use the Delta Factor and the Omega Attitude to create the life you want.

"The first wealth is health."
—Ralph Waldo Emerson

CHAPTER TEN

Where to From Here?

Congratulations! You're well on your way to Take Back Your Life. You've made excellent progress, and shown true courage in taking charge of your Outlook, Workout, and Nutrition in order to make a difference in your life.

Even so, setbacks will occur. If you prepare yourself for the fact that you may still 'backslide' from time to time, it's easier to get back on track. As you move forward, there will be times that you miss workouts because you've been sick or traveling. You'll eat some things that aren't optimum choices due to holidays, special occasions or lousy airport food courts.

Get back on track by OWNing your Outlook. Don't waste time beating yourself up over a few missed workouts or splurge dinners. Figure out what went wrong, fix it, and go on, getting back into the groove of your new, healthy life.

How will you handle times when you miss a workout, overdo on food, or fall into a funk? List several ways you've learned to pull yourself out of a misstep and get back on track.

....

....

....

....

....

....

Success begins with Outlook, so if your Outlook slips, the Workout and Nutrition may slip with it. That makes it essential for you stay focused on maintaining all that you've achieved and refuse to fall back into the "stinkin' thinkin'" that got you into trouble. You've learned a variety of ways to cheer yourself up, refocus on the positive, draw on the power of gratitude, and keep your eye on your goals.

Make your own list of ways you can keep your Outlook on track.

....

....

....

....

....

What are the most common reasons you slip up on your Workout? Crazy work hours? Travel? Responsibilities at home? Child care hassles? Whatever it is, realize that you can find ways to work around it. For example, resistance bands slip easily into a suitcase for on-the-go exercise. A few dumbbells at home, some jazzy music, and a flight of stairs can provide a good workout in a pinch.

What ideas can you come up with to rescue your Workout?

....

....

....

....

....

....

Think about the challenges that derail your Nutrition most often. Is it holiday get-togethers? Social events that revolve around food? A too-busy work or home schedule? Limited choices when traveling? Brainstorm some ways you can limit the damage. For example, can you carry a healthy snack in your purse while traveling? Get your social group to do something other than eat?

What are your ideas?

....

....

....

....

....

....

....

Make a promise to yourself that you will not allow yourself to go back to old, unhealthy ways of acting, eating or thinking. It's not just about the gym: you've fixed your Outlook, Workout, and Nutrition. If there are old hurts or patterns from your past that you need to work through, find a professional counselor and resolve the issues so that you are free to move on. You're worth it!

Write your promise to yourself here:

....

....

....

....

....

Now copy that promise onto several index cards and put the cards where you will see them several times a day to keep you motivated!

The health decisions you make at age 40 or 50 directly determine your quality of life at age 60, 70, and 80. Take a moment to envision what you want out of your life in your 'golden years' that will require health, energy, and a positive outlook. Notice how many things will be more enjoyable if you are in good shape, at a healthy weight, and in a positive mind frame.

Make your list here!

....

....

....

Now you know what to do. So do it! The time is gone for living in the past and wishing for the past to reappear so you can fix it. I know all too well, because I've been there. No one has ever been able to move forward with their eyes on the past, including myself.

Although we can't go back and make things better, we can change and gain control over what's happening now. Just keep in mind that new habits take time. Give yourself a break and believe it can happen for you too.

I can't say it enough . . . . **your outlook WILL determine your outcome!**

I am grateful that you chose me as your mentor to guide you through the best part of your life. I appreciate you and ask that you please keep the faith. I wish for you excellent health, incredible happiness, and phenomenal success!

"Things do not change; we change."
—Henry David Thoreau

APPENDIX ONE

Take Back your Life 90 day Goals

How do you want to look and feel three months from now?

1. ....

2. ....

3. ....

What are your eating, exercise, and lifestyle goals for the next 90 days?

1. ....

2. ....

3. ....

4. ....

What are some obstacles that might come up in the next 90 days?

1. ....

2. ....

3. ....

What are some strategies that can help you overcome these obstacles in the next 90 days?

1. ....
2. ....
3. ....

APPENDIX TWO

Tracking Sheet

Use this sheet to track your progress and stay motivated! Fill out the top when you first resolve to Take Back Your Life, and then update your measurements every month to record your achievements. Copy this page for your own use to have enough pages for each month you are on the program.

Day One: ....

Weight: ....

Measurements:

Waist...

Hips..

Chest ....

Upper arm ....

Thigh ....

Calf...

Body Fat: ....

Blood pressure:...

Blood sugar:..

Month:...

Weight: ....

Measurements:

Waist...

Hips ....

Chest ....

Upper arm ....

Thigh ....

Calf..

Body Fat: ....

Blood pressure:..

Blood sugar:...

Notes about progress and praise: (This might include increased flexibility, increased cardio endurance and increased strength-training capacity.) Record when you increase the weights you can lift and other notes of praise and motivation to yourself!

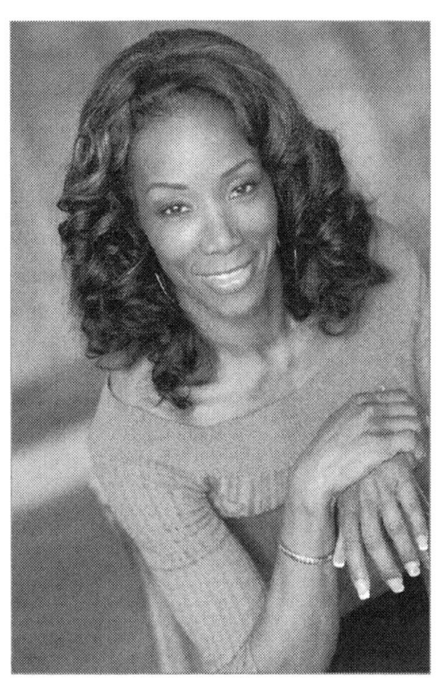

About the Author

WENDY IDA *(ee'da)* is a Nationally Certified Master Trainer, Nutrition Specialist and former Assistant Strength and Conditioning Coach for the LA Avengers football team.

Wendy is a Magazine Advice Columnist as well as a frequent guest on TV and talk radio. She has achieved international recognition via commercials, exercise videos and dozens of other appearances on Fox Sports Net, the Lifetime channel, TV1 and others. Wendy is a National Champion and five time winner of top trophy awards in the NPC Bodybuilding & Figure Championships.

She is Director of the Obesity Prevention Initiative (OPI) Program, with USC Norris Comprehensive Cancer Center, Kaiser Permanente, American Bio-Clinical Laboratories and the Real Men Cook Foundation.

Wendy grew up in New Jersey and has a bachelors degree in accounting, but decided to quit her 20 year Corporate Accounting job and start her fitness career at age 42 after she gained 50 pounds with the birth of her second child. Now her own personal journey from despair to reinventing herself as a premier personal trainer embodies her mantra that it is "never too late to take charge of your life".

Made in the USA
Lexington, KY
12 July 2019